Ketogenic Diet

The Ultimate Beginner's Guide to Ketogenic Diet

DOUGLAS H. MCCALLUM

The information herein is offered for informational purposes solely and is universal as so. The presentation of the information is without a contract or any type of guarantee assurance.

The trademarks that are used are without any consent, and the publication of the trademark is without permission or backing by the trademark owner. All trademarks and brands within this book are for clarifying purposes only and are the owned by the owners themselves, not affiliated with this document.

Table of Contents

Introduction

I want to thank you and congratulate you for downloading the book *Ketogenic Diet: The Ultimate Beginner's Guide to Ketogenic Diet.*

This book contains proven steps and strategies on how to use the ketogenic to your full advantage so that you may improve your overall health and wellness. The ketogenic diet offers a wide variety of mental and physical health benefits including weight loss, cholesterol control, blood pressure control, improved athletic performance, increased mental clarity, and blood glucose level maintenance. Whether you currently have a mental health condition that can be treated with the ketogenic diet or are simply looking for a diet that can help you to live healthier while avoiding the development of these conditions, the ketogenic diet is a great way to improve the way that your body works and feels!

This book contains information on what the ketogenic diet is, how it works, and the numerous health benefits that you can achieve with it. By reading this book and then utilizing the information that it contains, you will be able to help your body maintain better health and wellness. Whether your goals are to maintain healthy cholesterol levels, lower your blood pressure, or to lose weight; the ketogenic diet can help you to achieve those goals! By downloading and reading this eBook, we hope you are one step closer to achieving those goals and having a positive experience with the ketogenic diet. Most diet plans are tricky, and staying committed to a new diet can be difficult. This eBook helps make the details of the ketogenic diet simple to understand and easy to remember, this book also offers numerous tips to help you get the most from the ketogenic diet as well as various tips to help you stay committed!

Thanks again for downloading this book, I hope you enjoy it!

Chapter 1:

What is the Ketogenic Diet?

There are hundreds of available diet plans, and it seems like a new diet "fad" comes along each week. How do you decide which diet plan is right for you? They all claim to be successful, so it can be increasingly difficult to find a diet plan that is right for you (and it can be even more difficult to find the motivation to stick with it).

The ketogenic diet is a dietary concept that is easier to keep up with than some of the more complex diet plans. Unlike other strict diet plans, the ketogenic diet does not have a long and complex list of things that you cannot eat. The ketogenic diet also, unlike other diet programs, does not include a strict exercise regimen. The ketogenic diet keeps it pretty simple: focus on eating whole and healthy foods. That's it, that one statement sums up the whole ketogenic diet. Now, there are some smaller details to successfully adopting the ketogenic diet (of course) however these details all fall in line with the same summarizing statement. Exercise as much or as little as you like, and eat what you want as long as you are avoiding processed foods. Sugar and carbs are the only two "NO"'s on the ketogenic diet, and the "no carbs" rule is not a strict rule (rather, the ketogenic diet just aims to greatly reduce your carbohydrate intake).

Details of the Ketogenic Diet

The introductory paragraph sums up the basic ideas of the ketogenic diet, but there is admittedly a lot more to it. In a "picture perfect" world, an individual who is following the ketogenic diet strictly would have a daily diet plan that consists of 70% fat, 25% protein, and 5% carbs. This dietary plan supplies the body with healthy fats to burn for energy, protein to sustain good health, and a low intake of carbohydrates so that your body does not store away unhealthy (and unnecessary) weight in the form of fat reserves. While following the ketogenic diet, strive to eat mostly whole foods: whole foods, in this case, being foods with five or fewer ingredients. Processed foods are filled with artificial ingredients that are easier for your body to store away in fat reserves than to digest immediately, which is the why ketogenic diet aims to eliminate those from your daily food intake.

An easy way to determine what you should or should not be regularly consuming while on the ketogenic diet is to remember the "circle rule." When you go grocery shopping, try to stick to buying products from the outside circle of the grocery store. Most grocery stores have the outer walls stocked with fresh meats, produce, cheeses, and dairy. The circle rule (generally speaking) complies with the ketogenic diet because most grocery stores keep the foods you are avoiding eating stocked in the center aisles of the stores (sugars, grains, processed foods). By not allowing yourself to venture into the grocery store's center aisles, you will be skipping the opportunity to purchase frozen and processed foods. Make sure that you are buying the majority of your groceries from the produce, dairy, and fresh meat sections so that your ketogenic diet stays on track and your body truly benefits from your new diet plan. On the following page, we have compiled a brief chart to summarize the "goods" and "bads" of foods for this diet.

Good Foods	**Bad Foods**
- Meats	- Sugar (Soda, Candy, Juice)
- Seafood	- Grains & Starch (Bread, Rice, Potatoes)
- Eggs	- Processed Fats (Margarine)
- Above Ground Vegetables	- Beer
- Dairy (Full-Fat)	- Artificial Sweeteners
- Nuts & Seeds	- Legumes
- Olive Oil	- Dark Chocolate
- Coconut Oil/Flour	- Factory Farmed Fish/Pork

How the Ketogenic Diet Works

The ketogenic is centered around the body's natural, metabolic process of ketosis. When the body is in a state of ketosis, it is burning previously stored fat reserves in your body to get energy rather than using recently consumed sugars or carbohydrates as an energy source. The ketogenic diet is your body's evolved way of avoiding hypoglycemia. When you take part in a diet that eliminates carbohydrates, you also eliminate your body's primary energy source: glucose. Without glucose providing energy, your body will naturally sink to a state of hypoglycemia which can result in loss of motor skills and dizziness. To avoid hypoglycemia, your body switches to ketosis to obtain energy for daily activities. During ketosis, the liver burns stored fat to produce ketones. Ketones are fuel molecules that can act as an alternative source of energy instead of glucose. More traditional diet plans emphasize the importance of an elevated carbohydrate intake to have the energy required to increase your fitness plan. The ketogenic diet differs from traditional diet plans in numerous ways, the first being the since the ketogenic diet does not use glucose as an energy source the body must have an increase in fat intake rather than carbohydrates. Without the increased carbohydrate intake, the body's glucose levels fall which causes the release of previously stored triglycerides. Fatty acids then travel to the body's liver, where the liver produces ketones that will be used as the body's main energy source during a metabolic state of ketosis.

Many people consider the ketogenic diet to be a more natural dietary option than traditional diet plans, as the ketogenic diet does not ask your body to take glucose levels above a natural level to transform that glucose to a useable energy source. Instead of consuming an increased level of carbohydrates and greatly increasing the body's glucose levels, the ketogenic diet relies on natural metabolic processes to utilize the energy sources already stored within the body (fat) rather than adding more to it to find an energy source.

Chapter 2:

Ketogenic Diet Benefits

Ketogenic Diet & Glucose

The ketogenic diet offers multiple benefits to both mental and physical health. The health benefits that can be gained by the ketogenic diet are most commonly linked to the body's lack of glucose, as many health conditions are brought on or made worse by continued high levels of glucose or extreme sugar intake. In fact, one of the most commonly considered health benefits of the ketogenic diet is the diet plan's ability to control blood glucose levels (which can be vital in reversing type II diabetes, prediabetes, and multiple forms of cancer). The ketogenic is not used as an effective treatment for various forms of cancer, though it can aid in the prevention of cancer as many forms of cancer seem to use glucose as their number one fuel source. Various types of cancer cells and tumors use glucose as a primary energy source from which to grow and multiply. The ketogenic diet eliminates the consumption of glucose and greatly decreases an individual's daily consumption of carbohydrates which your body may transform to glucose to be used as energy. If glucose is not an available energy source within your body, you will be practically starving any existing cancer cells so that they not only stop growing but may deplete and shrink altogether due to a non-existent energy source. The ketogenic diet strives to increase your daily consumption of healthy and natural fatty acids, but cancer cells are unable to use these healthy fatty acids as an energy source. Since the ketogenic diet supplies your body with an available source of energy that cannot be utilized by cancer cells, your body will continue to function and burn weight while the cancer cells are starved off because of the lack of glucose in your body's bloodstream. We will go into a more in-depth discussion of the ketogenic diet's effects on cancerous cells later on in this book, the main idea to take away from this section is that the ketogenic diet is beneficial in controlling your body's blood glucose levels while offering an alternative and healthier primary energy source.

Ketogenic Diet & Heart Health

The ketogenic diet is a great way to improve your heart's health as well! The ketogenic diet helps to aid in blood pressure control as well as cholesterol control, two things that can greatly impact your risk of experiencing a heart attack or stroke. While the ketogenic diet can be great in helping to treat hypertension (high blood pressure) and high cholesterol, it is extremely important that the individual continues to regularly follow up with their physician in the case that additional treatment may be required depending on the severity of their condition. Increased glucose intakes in one's daily meal plans can lead to high cholesterol, high blood pressure, and coronary artery disease: three things which commonly cause heart attacks, heart failure, and stroke. By adopting a diet that eliminates the daily consumption of glucose (such as the ketogenic diet) you greatly reduce your risk of developing such heart problems. Previous studies have been performed which showed a positive correlation between the consumption of wheat and stroke, hypertensive heart disease, and cardiovascular disease. Since the ketogenic diet greatly reduces an individual's carbohydrate intake, wheat is almost eliminated with the diet which can result in a much lower risk of developing various cardiovascular diseases. Other studies have shown that individuals who regularly have diets consisting largely of carbohydrates are more likely to develop heart disease later in life. Eating excess amounts of carbohydrates increase your blood glucose levels, which increase your insulin levels and contribute to your overall insulin resistance. High blood sugar can also increase your risk of developing heart disease.

Ketogenic Diet & Weight Loss

Whether you have two-hundred pounds to lose or just twenty pounds, the ketogenic diet can help you do it. Not only does the ketogenic diet offer a fast and effective way in which to lose weight, but it is also a great form of healthy weight loss as well. With the ketogenic diet, you are training your body to eat the right kinds of healthy foods while drawing energy from what you have already stored (rather than taking in more glucose to use as an energy source). When your body is not constantly consuming a primary energy source (glucose) and is forced to burn previously stored fat for energy you will find yourself with the ability to shed weight in a fast and healthy way. The ketogenic diet is a healthy way for your body to lose weight because it eliminates the intake of sugar, which depletes the body's previously consumed storage of glycogen (sugar) and then forces the body to burn stored fat deposits to supply your cells with energy for daily activities. The ketogenic diet has also been known to be a healthy way in which to suppress your appetite, and it is more difficult to gain weight when you are eating less often (or less at regular meal times). An added benefit of the reduced hunger is the ketogenic diet's continuous energy supply. With your body burning glucose for energy, you only have as much energy as you consumed recently (which explains why athletes eat large meals consisting mainly of carbohydrates before a marathon or triathlon). The ketogenic diet forces your body to burn fat reserves for energy, which means your body always has a steady supply of energy available whenever you need it. Because the ketogenic diet offers a constant supply of energy, you will find yourself able to work out or remain active for longer periods of time on the ketogenic diet. While some diets teach that it is healthy to eat any fruits or vegetables, this is not so with the ketogenic diet. While on the ketogenic diet it is important to avoid most fruits because they tend to be high in glucose or natural sugars. Some vegetables such as those which are starchy or high in carbohydrates should also be avoided while on the ketogenic diet because your body uses the consumed carbohydrates and stores them as fat in your body. The best vegetables to eat while on the ketogenic diet are broccoli and green, leafy vegetables such as romaine lettuce and spinach. There are also multiple supplements that are available to be used in addition to a strict ketogenic diet so that you may experience the maximum amount of available health benefits, including accelerated weight loss (if weight loss if one of your current health goals and reasons for taking on the ketogenic diet). Suppressed hunger paired with increased energy and endurance make the ketogenic diet an ideal weight loss plan!

Ketogenic Diet & Mental Health

The majority of available diet plans can offer numerous physical health benefits, usually weight loss or weight management. Not many diet plans, however, can offer the benefit of improved mental health: that is where the ketogenic diet proves superior to other, more traditional diet plans. The ketogenic diet, and the metabolic process of ketosis in general are great for helping to eliminate brain fog, poor mental performance, and a general lack of productivity. Simply put, sugar is bad for brain function. Ketones, however, are great fuel for your brain! Ketones themselves are great in the treatment of neurodegenerative disorders such as Parkinson's disease, Alzheimer's disease, epilepsy, and a variety of age-related cognitive diseases. Many patients suffering from these ailments have the issue where their brains are unable to use enough glucose as a form of available energy to handle both perception and cognition, the ketogenic diet's use of ketones as a source of energy can assist in these problems where glucose itself is not sufficient as a primary energy source. Specifically, ketones have been shown to improve memory scores in Alzheimer's patients as well as improve various mild cognitive impairments seen in adults with advanced age.

Not only are ketones great for brain health and general function, but the increased fat consumption that makes up a ketogenic diet is also wonderful for improving brain function. The ketogenic emphasizes the importance of consuming healthy or natural fats such as fatty acids omega-3 and omega-6 (both are extremely crucial for optimal brain function and brain health). The majority of our brain tissue is made up of fatty acids, but the human body is unable to make these essential fatty acids on its own. Since our bodies cannot produce these fatty acids, we must obtain them through careful dietary habits: the ketogenic diet just happens to be a great way to regularly obtain these fatty acids in the form of natural fats. To consume the essential fatty acids for optimal brain health, be sure that you are including the right types of fat in your ketogenic diet. The best fats for obtaining omega-3s and omega-6s are coconut oil, fish, eggs, butter, avocados, and olive oil. Cooking oils such as vegetable oil and canola oil are not the natural or healthy fats that you are seeking to obtain to improve brain function on a ketogenic diet.

Ketogenic Diet & Epilepsy

Epilepsy is a condition that affects more than 300,000 children in the United States (these children being fifteen years old or younger). The children who suffer epilepsy are prone to seizures as well as other negative side effects stemming from epilepsy, and according to Mayo Clinic on in every four of these children also have an intellectual disability. Children who have been diagnosed with epilepsy also face a higher risk of developing anxiety, depression, and a variety of mood disorders. For some of these children with epilepsy, the seizures that they often experience cannot be eliminated by pharmaceutical therapy alone: this is where the ketogenic diet was born to shine. The ketogenic diet was developed in the 1920s at the Mayo Clinic and was developed to stimulate the body's natural metabolic state of ketosis by mimicking a fasting state within the body. Today, the ketogenic diet is still widely used to treat children who suffer from intractable seizures.

The good news about the ketogenic diet is that the families of these children are often able to adapt to their dietary changes relatively quickly and with ease. The ketogenic diet does restrict certain types of foods from consumption however it still offers a wide variety of options for families to incorporate into their daily meals. Children who are started on a ketogenic diet as a treatment plan for epilepsy are often started on a strict ketogenic diet while they are admitted to the hospital (usually for a three to five-day period) so that their body's response to the dietary changes can be noted and monitored (this also gives their parents adequate time to research and prepare for their new dietary needs and restrictions). Epilepsy can present itself through a variety of medical conditions including but not limited to tuberous sclerosis complex, infantile spasms, Rett syndrome, Dravet syndrome, GLUT-1 deficiency, and Doose syndrome. The ketogenic diet can help to treat the epilepsy of children whose seizures have not been able to be treated effectively using common varieties of anti-seizure medications.

The results of the ketogenic diet show that it is extremely helpful as a natural form of treatment for various seizure disorders including epilepsy. Over 50% children who were placed on a strict ketogenic diet saw at least a 50% decrease in the number of seizures that they experienced. A much lower percentage of children (an estimated 15%) who were placed on the ketogenic diet as a treatment plan for seizure disorders were also able to experience the result of being seizure free without the help of medications. Anyone who has a history or current diagnosis of epilepsy or a related condition should consult their doctor before beginning a ketogenic diet. The ketogenic diet is a healthy treatment option for most people and may be regularly monitored by a dietician after being prescribed by your primary care doctor. While the ketogenic diet was able to help some epilepsy patients stay seizure free without the use of traditional medications, some patients may still need to use reduced dosages of anti-seizure medications while on the ketogenic diet to fully benefit and eliminate seizures.

Ketogenic Diet & Cancer

While the ketogenic diet does not claim to be an effective "cure" for cancer, it has been used as both a form of treatment and prevention for numerous variations of cancer. The ketogenic diet is currently under investigation as a form of treatment for cancers because it eliminates the consumption of sugars for the participating individuals, this may work as a treatment for various types of cancers because cancer cells and tumors rely on glucose for energy. Dr. Thomas Seyfried (and other cancer research professionals) has found that cancer cells obtain their main source of energy from the fermentation of glutamine (an amino acid). The ketogenic diet may offer an effective form of treatment for various cancers because it effectively starves the cancer cells or tumors since it eliminates glucose from your body. Your body's natural metabolic state of ketosis has been proven to deplete your body's fat storage, but can ketosis deplete the energy supply that fuels cancer cells too?

Cancer cells are unlike our body's normal cells in numerous ways, however, one of the key differences is that cancer cells have up to ten times more insulin receptors on their surface than our body's normal cells do. With an excessive amount of insulin receptors, cancer cells can inhale glucose at an alarmingly high rate. Basically, this means that so long as you are consuming glucose, you will also be allowing cancer cells to gorge themselves on that glucose which will result in them thriving and growing within your body. Studies have shown that cancer patients with the lowest blood sugar levels also tend to have the highest survival rates, this adds to the evidence that the ketogenic diet may be a viable option for various cancer treatments.

The ketogenic diet may work as a form of cancer treatment in two ways: the ketogenic diet eliminates the primary fuel source of cancer cells while increasing our body's supply of a fuel source which the cancer cells are unable to utilize. Think of it this way: imagine that a cancerous tumor is a car. The ketogenic diet eliminates any form of gasoline (glucose) for the car (cancerous tumor) to use as fuel but instead offers an abundant supply of water (fat) to be used as fuel. Cars do not run on water, just as cancer cells cannot survive off of fatty acids. The ketogenic diet eliminates cancer's primary fuel source (glucose) while increasing the amount of fat which we provide for our bodies to turn into an alternate energy source (ketones).

Intermittent fasting has been shown to be an effective technique for increasing the production of ketones, which will simultaneously starve cancer cells at an accelerated rate. Some studies have also shown that late-stage cancer patients can maximize the weakening of their cancer cells by taking on a lemon water cleanse for a set duration of five to seven days. By choosing to participate in a 20 hour fast (only offering a feeding window of four hours each day), you are maximizing the number of ketones which your body will be forced to produce as fuel, thereby weakening your cancer cells as much as you possibly can be depleting their primary energy source of glucose.

Ketogenic Diet & Lyme Disease

Diet can be a very influential part of someone's daily life when dealing with Lyme disease. When it comes to the effective treatment of Lyme disease, it is essential to try to boost your body's immune system through whatever means possible (the ketogenic diet is a great diet for naturally boosting your body's immune system). Not only does the ketogenic diet help boost your body's immune system, but the intermittent fasting that is so essential to the success of the ketogenic diet is key in rebooting your body's immune system as well as maintaining your body's metabolic state of ketosis. There are several claims that diets such as the ketogenic diet that restrict or eliminate the regular intake of carbohydrates can be an effective form of treatment for Lyme disease. The ketogenic diet has not been proven to be a cure for Lyme disease itself, though it has been shown to alleviate many of the symptoms brought on by Lyme disease. Those who are suffering from Lyme disease often experience inflammation throughout their body. Consuming an increased amount of healthy "good" fat can greatly reduce inflammation throughout the body which can also aid in the reduction of joint stiffness, joint pain, and arthritis. Taking on the ketogenic diet and consuming an increased amount of fat will help the healthy bacteria or microflora found in your gut to thrive. The good bacteria found in your gut help your immune system to function at peak performance, which will result in your immune system being able to deal with fighting Lyme disease in a more effective and healthier manner. Another major symptom felt by individuals with Lyme disease is the disease's effect on their nervous system. It is common knowledge that the brain is a key part of the body's central nervous system. By adopting the ketogenic diet, you are providing your body with omega-3 fatty acids that are essential for optimal brain health (something that is key in dealing with Lyme disease and its effects on your body's central nervous system).

Ketogenic Diet & Oxygen Toxicity Seizures

Central nervous system oxygen toxicity is a condition in which the individual experiences seizures, loss of coordination, and muscle spasms. This condition often affects Navy SEAL divers as well as scuba divers because they use enriched oxygen gas masks from which they inhale elevated partial pressures of oxygen. Oxygen toxicity complications have also been found to affect individuals who use supplemental oxygen for various medical conditions (including premature infants). A recent article published in the American Journal of Physiology shows that the utilization of a ketogenic diet may prevent central nervous system toxicity. Ketogenic diets can help with central nervous system toxicity because the ketogenic diet provides the body with increased amounts of ketones and ketones have been found to be neuroprotective in that they help our brains to better preserve energy in situations of oxidative stress (such as hyperbaric oxygen therapy and special operations diving done by our military forces).

Ketogenic Diet & Acne

While the various health benefits offered by those who adopt the ketogenic diet are still being researched, one of the commonly known benefits of the ketogenic diet is the diet's ability to help reduce acne. Acne can be caused by the consumption of excess amounts of sugar and insulin resistance, two things that are eliminated by the ketogenic diet since the diet itself strives to avoid all sources of glucose. Without the regular consumption of glucose, you are practically starving acne as a way to eliminate it. Some studies have also shown that diet plans that are low in carbohydrates can also greatly help in the reduction of acne (which would also explain why the ketogenic diet helps eliminate acne since the diet is very low carb). Many individuals who have practiced a strict ketogenic diet for multiple weeks find that their skin is often restored to a state of being almost unnaturally flawless. The ketogenic diet can greatly decrease the amount of oil which your skin produces, which means less oil available to clog your skin's pores and cause irritating acne as a result. While the ketogenic diet does not offer an overnight cure for acne, many individuals who have undertaken the ketogenic diet saw dramatic improvements in their skin condition after a few weeks of a strictly ketogenic diet.

Ketogenic Diet & Alzheimer's

The ketogenic diet's positive results as a partial treatment for Alzheimer's may be largely based on the added omega-3 fatty acids that our body gains by participating in the ketogenic diet. Omega-3 fatty acids are vital for optimal brain function and brain health, which could be why the ketogenic diet may be used to relieve some of the symptoms experienced by those who are living with Alzheimer's disease. Multiple studies have been performed that show a direct correlation between mental health declination and insulin resistance. The body's natural metabolic state of ketosis helps our body to increase our insulin sensitivity which decreases our blood glucose levels (done by restricted carbohydrate intake as well as the elimination of sugar consumption) that can greatly increase our brain health and performance.

A small study (consisting of twenty patients) was performed to outline the correlation between ketosis and patients with cognitive impairments such as Alzheimer's disease. Half of the patients were given a placebo, and the other half were given a medium chain triglyceride (MCT). The patients who were given the medium chain triglyceride were shown to have increase ketone levels after just 90 minutes, these patients also showed greater improvements in their memory. This study shows a positive correlation between the body's state of ketosis and optimal brain function. As if this study was not adequate evidence between the ketogenic diet and Alzheimer's, a similar and larger study was performed on 150 patients five years later. All 150 patients had been diagnosed with a mild case of Alzheimer's, and a number of patients in the study were given a ketogenic supplement to be monitored as a part of the study. The patients who were given the ketogenic supplement should cognitive improvements a full 45 days after the start of the study, offering further evidence that the body's natural state of ketosis is beneficial to brain health.

There are several health conditions that may increase an individual's risk for developing Alzheimer's disease, some of these conditions include diabetes, high cholesterol, and inflammation. If you do not believe that the ketogenic diet can be a beneficial form of treatment for Alzheimer's or other cognitive disabilities, consider that the ketogenic diet is commonly used to treat the conditions that can lead to the development of Alzheimer's. The ketogenic diet can effectively treat diabetes, joint inflammation, and high cholesterol. In treating these various health conditions with a ketogenic diet, an individual can also greatly reduce their risk for developing Alzheimer's disease.

Chapter 3:

How to Keto

After you have done some reading on the ketogenic diet and have decided that you can benefit greatly from it (everyone can), the next step is to adopt the ketogenic diet as your dietary plan and get started! As with any new diet that asks you to alter your daily meal plan, starting a new diet can be difficult. Like most people, you may find yourself very motivated to start a new diet in the beginning but begin to lose that motivation to stay committed to it after a week or so. Make sure that you have the information and tools available to you that you will need to stay committed to the ketogenic diet. Information is the most important tool that you can have when beginning a new diet, so we have outlined numerous key points of the ketogenic diet below including exercise tips, the "dos" and "don'ts" of food consumption, and tips on fasting for the ketogenic diet. The information outlined below is outlined and compiled to make your experience with the ketogenic as easy and beneficial to you as possible!

Food *Dos* and *Don'ts*

The ketogenic diet may be one of the easiest diet plans to stay committed to simply because the list of foods that you are still allowed to eat every day is pretty extensive. You are still able to keep a healthy diet with a wide variety of food options on the ketogenic diet, unlike other diets that may greatly limit what you are allowed to eat (making it much more difficult to stay committed). On the ketogenic diet, you are encouraged to eat proteins, and there aren't many restrictions on what types of meat are okay to eat. Allowable meats on the ketogenic diet range from beef to seafood and include beef, chicken, duck, pork, turkey, cured meats, sausages, bacon (low carb, low sugar), and seafood. The list of encouraged seafood on the ketogenic diet includes salmon, tuna, squid, scallops, muscles, prawns, haddock, anchovies, trout, sardines, and mackerel.

The ketogenic diet allows and encourages you to enjoy eggs as often as you would like, and in any way that you would like! Drinks on the ketogenic diet are fair so long as they remain unsweetened. Like with any diet, it is ideal to drink water (and lots of it). The ketogenic diet also allows for one to drink tea and coffee daily, so long as you avoid adding any dairy or sugar to them (cream is okay). As with other diets, the ketogenic diet wants vegetables to be your best friend! Most vegetables are great for this diet, so long as they have been grown above ground.

The ketogenic diet wants for you to consume large amounts of vegetables such as asparagus, cauliflower, cucumber, kale, green beans, broccoli, Brussel sprouts, cabbage, peppers, mushrooms, olives, lettuce, radishes, spinach, tomatoes, snow peas, onions, and pumpkin. Avoid vegetables that are starchy or grown below ground such as potatoes and carrots. Seeds are a great way to snack on the ketogenic diet, as they offer a source of healthy fat. Chia, flax, sesame, pumpkin, and even sunflower seeds are allowable and encouraged snack options with the ketogenic diet. You can also enjoy a variety of flours (almond, coconut, and hazelnut) as well as nuts (almonds, hazelnuts, pecans, pine nuts, and walnuts) on the ketogenic diet. Dairy is allowable so long as it is full fat and low sugar: think of options like cream, butter, blue cheese, cream cheese, feta cheese, Greek yogurt, and parmesan cheese.

Now for the list of "NO" foods, the least favourite part of any diet plan (though luckily with the ketogenic diet, the list of NO foods is a lot shorter than the list of allowable foods). On the ketogenic diet, try to avoid the following vegetables: corn, peas, carrots, and potatoes. Avoid eating fruits of all kinds, as these can be high in sugars, except for special occasions when a small serving of fruit is okay. Avoid various grains such as barley, buckwheat, quinoa, pinto beans, red beans, soy, and all types of rice. Carbohydrates are not included in the ketogenic diet, remember that the whole idea of this diet is to eliminate the consumption of carbs. Eliminating carbohydrates from your daily meal plan means not eating any bread, bagels, cake, candy, brownies, chips, oats, pasta, crackers, cookies, cupcakes, pastries, popcorn, pizza, rolls, tortillas, or tortilla chips. Drinks that are off limits with the ketogenic diet include alcohol, sweetened coffee, juice, sodas, and sweetened teas. It is also a good idea to avoid anything that is "diet" or artificially sweetened, gum included.

There are a wide variety of ketogenic approved diets available online as well as in books that offer a great way to stick to the list of allowable ketogenic foods while still allowing you to experience a variety of foods while dieting. Chapter five of this book also offers more than a dozen delicious recipes for you to try while you practice the ketogenic diet!

Keto Exercise Tips

There are four types of exercise that one may choose to practice during their experience with the ketogenic diet. While the ketogenic diet does not include a strict workout plan, these four exercises will work well with the diet itself while offering numerous health benefits to your mind and body. For maximum health benefits, be sure to try each of the four exercise types multiple times each week so that you do not find yourself becoming bored with the same exercise each day.

The first exercise type that is encouraged on the ketogenic diet is stability exercise. Stability exercises include activities such as core training, planking, ball exercises and other balance promoting activities. Stability exercises work to improve your core strength, which is great for the following benefits: toning abdominal muscles, reducing the risk of injury, improving balance, improving posture, aligning the spine, and improving athletic performance.

The second exercise type that is encouraged on the ketogenic diet is flexibility exercise. Flexibility exercises include activities such as stretching and yoga. The most common and obvious benefit of yoga or other stretching exercises is the increased flexibility that your body will begin to gain after. Yoga can also be very beneficial in improving balance, core strength, and endurance as these exercises ask your body to hold very still in (sometimes unnatural) poses for minutes at a time. Stretching is an essential pre-workout practice to avoid serious injuries such as muscle strains or tears. Yoga is also extremely beneficial for stress relief and mood elevation.

The third exercise type that is encouraged on the ketogenic diet is anaerobic exercises. Anaerobic exercises are defined as short but highly intense exercises lasting anywhere from a few seconds to two minutes. Anaerobic exercise activities include sprinting, jumping rope, weight lifting, isometrics, and biking. These various anaerobic exercise activities offer numerous physical benefits to your body including an increase in muscle strength.

The fourth and final exercise type that is encouraged on the ketogenic diet is aerobic exercises. Aerobic exercises include activities such as cardio workouts and running. Aerobic exercise activities are a great way to improve your body's general health as they help to lower cholesterol, improve the immune system, lower blood pressure, burn fat (weight loss), and reduce your risk for type 2 diabetes.

Ketogenic Diet & Fasting

Fasting can be an extremely beneficial part of any diet, but this is especially true for individuals who are taking part in the ketogenic diet. Some of the most common health benefits of fasting are the purging of cancerous or precancerous cells, improved sensitivity to insulin, enhanced cognitive effects, and a decrease in fat tissue (resulting in weight loss).

People who are discussing fasting while taking part in the ketogenic diet are usually referring specifically to intermittent fasting, a type of fasting that works particularly well with the ketogenic diet. Intermittent fasting means that you only allow yourself to eat during a previously set time period. For example, you may decide that your fasting period is from 7pm to 11 am, and your "feeding" window is from 11am to 7pm. This schedule for intermittent fasting would mean that each day for you consists of an 8-hour feeding window and a 16-hour fasting period. Beginning fasting may be difficult, but after you have been fasting for a period of several weeks, you may find yourself able to shrink your feeding window to only last five or six hours rather than eight or nine hours.

Fasting can be a difficult habit to get into, though the ketogenic diet can make the beginning phases of fasting a bit easier because the ketogenic diet's high-fat content leaves you feeling full from the consumption of less foods. The first step to fasting for many people is the act of meal skipping, as this gets your body used to going from prolonged periods without consuming foods. For example: if you are considering beginning fasting by meal skipping, you may decide to stick to the routine of skipping breakfast on weekdays or skipping lunch on weekends.

When fasting, it is important that you still remember to keep your body hydrated. During your fasting periods, it is best to drink water, unsweetened tea, or black coffee while abstaining from food consumption until you come up to your next feeding window.

The health benefits of fasting are plenty, and fasting can offer additional benefits in making your adoption of the ketogenic diet successful. Fasting helps an individual to deplete their body of previously stored glycogen in an expedient manner, which can help your body to enter a state of ketosis more quickly. For optimal results, beginning fasting two to three days before beginning your ketogenic diet (this will give your body the chance to begin reducing its glycogen storage). Fasting can not only help you to begin the metabolic stage of ketosis faster, but fasting can also help you to lose weight at a faster rate. By fasting, your body begins depleting its glycogen stores and breaking down fat to use for energy more quickly, both resulting in weight loss. Fasting also helps you to lose weight because you are more likely to consume a smaller amount of food in your restricted feeding window than you would normally throughout the day.

Intermittent fasting means that you are only allowing yourself to consume foods for a restricted time period during each day, which will result in your consuming less calories each day without having to really try to. When you are intermittent fasting, you do not have to "count calories," and you can eat as much of the approved foods as you wish during your feeding window. The ketogenic diet consists largely of foods with a high-fat content, so you are more likely to feel full after eating just once or twice during your feeding window (as opposed to eating three meals and two snacks throughout the day as you normally might). Since you are likely to consume less calories during intermittent fasting, it is obvious why this dietary technique may help an individual to quickly lose weight.

Fasting helps an individual's body to begin the metabolic state of ketosis more quickly, which is extremely beneficial in improving one's mental clarity. Your brain functions in a much better way when it is fueled by ketones, which can be great in helping you to maintain focus and improve mental performance. The dietary practice of fasting will help to improve your overall health and wellness by supporting muscle growth, improving metabolism, reducing inflammation, improving insulin sensitivity, and improving one's longevity.

Staying Keto Committed!

Starting a new diet plan can be hard to do, but perhaps the most difficult part of any diet is staying committed. Most people start new diets with a ton of motivation behind them, but slowly lose this motivation after just a few short days or weeks. Consider the last time you started a diet, are you still dieting? Why not? How long did your last diet last? Speaking from experience, it is very easy to think about the various foods that you are "missing out on" while dieting, which can lead to a congratulatory "cheat day." When you have been on a strict new diet for three weeks, it is easy to tell yourself that you are doing great and you deserve a cheat day. Just one day to eat whatever you want, then you'll go back to dieting like a champ: easy right? Wrong! One misstep on your diet can derail your whole diet because it is so easy to take a cheat day but only that much more difficult to get back into dieting afterward. So how do you stay motivated and committed while adopting a new diet, such as the ketogenic diet? Below we have compiled and outlined a number of various tips that will be able to help you stay committed to your ketogenic diet!

1. Don't Try to Do It Alone: Our first tip for staying motivated or committed on the ketogenic diet is to try to avoid doing it alone. It can be very difficult to start a new diet, and beginning or sticking to the ketogenic diet can be more difficult if you force yourself to watch your friends consuming soda and pasta for every meal. If you start the diet with a friend or even have someone who wants to try it out with you after you have already started, you will have a much easier time staying committed to your dietary goals. Having a "diet buddy" means that you have someone to motivate and also get motivation from. Whenever you are having a moment of doubt or temptation, you have your diet buddy to remind you of your goals. Having someone on the same diet who knows what you are going through also gives you someone to communicate with about your struggles and successes on the ketogenic diet because they have the same experiences!

2. *Keep Reading:* Our second tip for keeping your motivation for the ketogenic diet going after you have started is to keep reading up on the ketogenic diet itself. I am sure that you have done adequate research about the ketogenic diet beforehand, and having armed yourself with that necessary information to be successful, you are now ready to begin. Keep reading up on the ketogenic diet, it's "dos" and "don'ts," and the ketogenic lifestyle after you have started. By continuing your research as you take on the ketogenic diet, you will find yourself more motivated by the continuous new information and will always be learning about more benefits of the ketogenic diet (which will help you stay committed to keto). Think of it this way, you would obviously learn how to fire a gun before heading off to war: but why go to war unarmed?

3. *Develop a Morning Routine:* If you start each day on a positive and motivated note, you are more likely to get through the day without failure. Prepare yourself for the challenges and temptations that you may face during the day ahead because you are more likely to fail by challenges that come to you as a surprise rather than the ones which you have prepared yourself to face. Develop a morning routine that will help you to begin each day on a more positive note. Try to wake up well ahead of time each morning so that you have time to reflect on your successes and relax before attempting to accomplish anything or facing anything stressful. Exercise is a great way to begin each morning because it awakens your body and helps to release "good feeling" chemicals and hormones in your brain. You can also try to begin each morning by finding a motivational quote to return to throughout the day to stay committed, the internet and Pinterest have millions of positive, inspirational, and motivation quotes (thousands are even diet related)!

4. Keep a Journal: A great way to help you stay committed to a new diet is to keep a journal outlining your progress that has been made so far on that diet. If you have physical evidence in front of you, in your own word, of how far you have come, then you are less likely to relapse and fall back to your own poor health habits. A journal can be used as a valuable tool on your ketogenic diet journey, as a journal would provide a way for you to look back on your previous successes anytime that you find yourself in doubt. In your journal, be sure to keep track of things like weight loss, days when you find yourself feeling better than usual, and times when you have faced the temptation to quit or take a break from your ketogenic diet but overcame temptation and stuck with it.

5. Stay Hydrated: Like with any diet, it is extremely important to be sure that you keep well-hydrated while on the ketogenic diet. Staying well hydrated not only offers numerous health benefits but staying hydrated can help you stay committed to your new journey with the ketogenic diet as well. Staying hydrated by drinking a lot of water will help your body to achieve that feeling of being "full" more often, which will mean you are less likely to experience extreme cravings for foods that you should be avoiding on the ketogenic diet. Drinking excess amounts of water instead of choosing soda will also help you to feel like you are making progress on your diet which can help you stay motivated and committed. The last and perhaps the most obvious way in which water helps you to stay committed to your diet is the way in which it affects your brain. Your brain cannot function at peak performance if your body is not well hydrated, and when your brain is not performing optimally, you are more likely to make poor decisions.

6. Remember the Starting Line: After you have been practicing the ketogenic diet for a few weeks and you are beginning to lose motivation, remember where you were when you started this diet. Ask yourself some of the following questions: why did you start the ketogenic diet? What were your goals for the ketogenic diet? Has the ketogenic diet helped you to achieve any of your health goals or have you felt better physically since beginning the ketogenic diet? Remember how you felt when you started the ketogenic diet and took some time to reflect on your successes with the diet so far as well as how far you have come since beginning the ketogenic diet: this will help you to remain positive and motivated about your dietary practices.

7. Set Specific Goals: Part of staying committed to any diet is being able to visualize and work towards specific, previously set goals. By setting goals for yourself, small and large, you are creating several "finish lines" for yourself. In achieving even a small goal (like staying on the diet for one month) and crossing that finish line, you will feel a sense of accomplishment that will motivate you to continue forward in achieving more goals. Consider this: is it easier for you to achieve the specific goal of losing five pounds or the general goal of "I want to be skinny"? Specific goals are much easier to achieve and are not subjective, so they are also easier to be proud of. General opinions are often based on opinion: skinny to you may not be skinny to other people, and developing healthier eating habits may still be viewed as unhealthy to others who are stricter about their dietary practices. Specific goals help you to narrow your focus and achieve your dietary goals in a more precise, and even expedient manner.

8. Clear the Pantry: This last and final helpful tip to staying committed to the ketogenic diet is perhaps one of the first that you should accomplish. One of the first things you should do when beginning the ketogenic diet is to clear out your pantry. When starting the ketogenic diet, throw away all of the "bad" foods that you have in your house because you are less likely to cave and eat junk food if you have to go out and get it first. We have all heard the phrase "out of sight, out of mind," and that can heavily apply to our dietary practices too. You are more likely to find yourself cheating with a bag of chips if they are staring at you from the pantry every day, however if they are nowhere to be found you are more likely to forget about their existence and make healthier food choices. Not only should you clear out your pantry at the beginning of your diet, but make sure to do a "clean sweep" on a weekly basis to help you stay committed as well.

Doing a regular clear out of your pantry is especially important if you do not live alone, as there may be other people bringing the exact foods that you are trying to avoid into your home. While we understand that you cannot just throw away your roommate's food, you can ask them to keep the unhealthy foods to their room or in an area away from where your food is kept so that you are not likely to fail on your ketogenic diet.

Chapter 4:

Ketogenic Supplements

While the ketogenic diet does offer dozens of health benefits on its own, there are ways in which to maximize the benefits that you will see by adopting the ketogenic diet. If you begin and remain committed to the ketogenic diet, you are sure to see numerous improvements to your physical and mental health: however, these benefits can be emphasized and seen in a more expedient manner if you utilize certain supplements to aid in your ketogenic diet goals. This chapter contains information about various supplements that will be able to help you maximize the health benefits which you can receive from the ketogenic diet.

Vitamin D: There are currently more than one billion people in the world who have a vitamin D deficiency, which can lead to some serious negative health effects. Vitamin D may not help specifically with the bodily process of ketosis, but vitamin D is essential to various body functions such as immunity, muscle function, and calcium absorption. If you are wondering how you can be sure to consume an adequate amount of vitamin D while on the ketogenic diet, you do not need to worry because vitamin D is found in several key keto foods such as mushrooms, fatty fish, fish oils, and egg yolks. While there are several ketogenic approved foods from which you can get vitamin D, the best way to make sure you are giving your body vitamin D is to get it naturally from the sun. This can be a great time to "kill two birds with one stone" by exercising outside while simultaneously absorbing vitamin D into your body from the sun. Exercising outside not only exposes your body to much-needed vitamin D and allows for a chance for exercise, but it also gives you the chance to breathe in fresh air and relax as you spend some time in the great outdoors.

L- Glutamine: L-Glutamine is a supplement that can benefit you while you are doing the ketogenic diet because it is an amino acid, but it acts as an antioxidant for your body. L-Glutamine is a great supplement to take on the ketogenic diet if you are an individual who is very active because excessive exercise tends to result in the depletion of your body's natural glutamine storage (which can release free radicals or toxins in your body). You may also not be consuming enough antioxidants while on the ketogenic diet because the ketogenic diet requires that you avoid several antioxidant-rich fruits and vegetables. Supplementing the ketogenic diet with an antioxidant like L-Glutamine can help to prevent cellular damage as well as help with muscle recovery and boosting your body's immune system. By taking a supplement that helps with muscle recovery, you will also find yourself needing less time for your body to recover between workouts which will maximize your ability to increase muscle strength, stamina, and endurance.

Electrolytes: Starchy fruits and vegetables are a great and natural source of electrolytes, so it is understandable that one may worry that they are not consuming enough electrolytes while on the ketogenic diet. One way to eliminate this concern is to take an electrolyte supplement while on the ketogenic diet so that you do not have to worry about reducing electrolytes by reducing your overall carbohydrate consumption. There are several different forms of electrolytes, two of the more common electrolytes are magnesium and calcium. Both calcium and magnesium help to reduce anxiety and stress, for this reason, they have come to be known as the "calming electrolytes." These "calming electrolytes" can be extremely beneficial in helping you keep calm as you may experience mild levels of stress in transitioning to a low carbohydrate diet. Electrolytes are also key in aiding with overcoming the commonly experienced "keto flu." The "keto flu" is a series of symptoms that are sometimes felt by those who are newly adapting to the ketogenic diet. The "keto flu" often includes feelings of fatigue, dizziness, headaches, nausea, and muscle cramping. Many of the symptoms of keto flu can be made worse by low levels of electrolytes, and taking an additional electrolyte supplement may help to weaken or even eliminate keto flu symptoms.

MCT Oil: The abbreviation MCT stands for medium chain triglycerides. Medium chain triglycerides (MCT's) are a foundation of fat molecule (fatty acid) which can be found in many everyday food sources such as yogurt, cheese, butter, and certain oils. Medium chain triglycerides can be used as an energy source right away, which makes them slightly better than other types of fatty acids. Medium chain triglycerides are converted to ketones and used for fuel almost immediately, unlike other fatty acids that may take longer to metabolize (causing them to be stored as fat rather than used immediately as an energy source). The regular consumption of medium chain triglycerides helps to keep your body in a constant state of fat burning by offering a continuous energy source. Coconut oil is a great source of medium chain triglycerides (we'll discuss that later), but there are several benefits of taking an MCT oil over just coconut oil. MCT oil is easier for your body to utilize over coconut oil containing MCT because the medium chain triglycerides have already been separated from the other nutrients found in coconut oil. Since your body does not have to separate the medium chain triglycerides from any other ingredients, it can use them for energy in a more expedient manner. Medium chain triglyceride supplements will also help you to meet your daily fat requirements for remaining in a state of ketosis. Medium chain triglyceride supplements are easy to add to your daily ketogenic diet because you can easily mix them in with your favorite keto friendly smoothies, milkshakes, teas, and coffees.

Creatine: The first thing to know about creatine is that creatine is an amino acid. Amino acids, including creatine, play a vital role in muscle contractions as well as energy production. Creatine is an important supplement to utilize when it comes to exercise and fitness plans, as many athletes and bodybuilders rely on this supplement to building lean muscle mass and increasing levels of endurance. Creatine is an amino acid that is produced naturally by our bodies, though our bodies do produce lower levels of creatine as we age. Amino acids can help you (as an athlete) to achieve occasional bursts of energy and speed during your workouts. If you are an individual who strives to exercise regularly, you can benefit from concentrated doses of amino acids in the form of an added creatine supplement. Some of the basic health benefits that can be obtained by adding creatine supplements to your ketogenic diet are weight loss, improved athletic performance, building lean muscle mass, and increased muscle strength. You will also benefit from creatine supplements because creatine has been shown to help muscles recover in a more expedient manner during exercise and between workouts.

Fish Oil: On a ketogenic diet, it is extremely important to maintain a healthy omega 3:6 ratio. It is very difficult to be getting enough of the necessary fish oils simply from consuming fish, though you can be sure to get enough fish oils by adding a fish oil supplement to your diet. Fish oil supplements contain various oils that are obtained from the skin and liver of fatty fish species such as mackerel, sardines, and salmon. Fish oil supplements aid your body by providing it with vital omega-3 fatty acids that help to protect against heart disease (as well as various other health conditions). There are three types of omega-3 fatty acids: alpha-linolenic acid (ALA), docosahexaenoic acid (DHA), and eicosapentaenoic acid (EPA). ALA can be found in various ketogenic diet-friendly foods such as chia seeds, walnuts, and some oils; however, EPA and DHA can only be obtained from the consumption of fish oil supplements (or the fatty fish from which they are derived). As important as omega-3 fatty acids are, our bodies do not produce them naturally (which means you must consume fish or fish oil supplements to supply your body with them). Fish oil supplements are a great tool in ketogenic diets because they reduce the level so f triglycerides in your body (triglycerides are fat molecules in the bloodstream that store energy for your body to use at a later time).

7 Keto DHEA: 7 Keto DHEA is a varied metabolite of dehydroepiandrosterone (DHEA) that is produced by your adrenal glands as well as your brain. 7 Keto DHEA can help aid in the production of other hormones that help in increasing lean muscle mass and fat burning because it acts as a growth hormone. There have been studies that suggest that 7 Keto DHEA also has the ability to increase the activity of your body's thermogenic liver enzymes (these enzymes help your body to burn fatty acids more efficiently), which can help you to lose both weight and fat while you are on the ketogenic diet. 7 Keto DHEA is an essential supplement for the ketogenic diet if you want to boost your metabolism (in a natural way) and/or if you are looking to lose both weight and fat.

Perfect Keto: Perfect Keto is a ketogenic diet supplement that is offered as a powdered drink mix that can be added to your ketogenic friendly beverages (water, teas, smoothies). Perfect Keto supplies your body with exogenous ketones not produced by your body (your body produces endogenous ketones) which provide you with ketones that can be burned as an energy source immediately. These exogenous ketones can be burned as an immediate fuel source even when your body is not currently in a state of ketosis. There are people who greatly benefit from the Perfect Keto supplement even when they are not following a strict ketogenic diet because they still benefit from the healthy energy source provided by ketones. The Perfect Keto supplement helps your body to experience many of the same benefits offered by the ketogenic diet such as improved athletic performance, mental focus, fat burning, long-lasting energy, and accelerated weight loss. The Perfect Keto supplement can also help your body to stay in a state of ketosis, which will prolong the other numerous benefits offered by the ketogenic diet. If you are following a strict ketogenic diet but have exceeded your carbohydrate intake limit for the day, the Perfect Keto supplement will help your body get back into ketosis.

Coconut Oil: Coconut oil, as previously discussed, is a wonderful source of medium chain triglycerides (MCT's). Medium chain triglycerides make up roughly sixty percent of coconut oil's fat content, making it extremely healthy for your body. Coconut oil is an easy supplement to incorporate into your diet: you can melt it to a liquid state and mix it in with your smoothies, or you can also use it as a cooking oil since it has a mild flavor to it. Coconut oil can also add a healthy topping option if drizzled with beef, chicken, veggies, or even fish. The medium chain triglycerides that are found in coconut oil can act as a vital source of energy for your muscles and brain.

Caffeine: While caffeine itself may not be a key part to successful participation in the ketogenic diet, keep caffeine as a (minimal) part of your diet can help you to remain motivated to achieve your other health and ketogenic goals. When you switch from a high carbohydrate diet to a high-fat diet, your brain is going to require some time to become accustomed to its new energy source. While your body is making this transition, you may feel sluggish or "off" for a few days, and this is where caffeine comes in as a beneficial supplement. You can increase your caffeine intake by drinking more (black) coffee or by taking a caffeine supplement such as a fat burner or pre-workout supplement. Until your brain gets used to using ketones as a primary energy source, you may find yourself lacking the motivation to workout (or even just to stick to your ketogenic diet). By increasing your caffeine intake slightly, you can help your brain power through the "lag" phase that your body will experience as you switch from using glycogen as a primary energy source to using ketones as a primary energy source. Caffeine can help you to remain focused and motivated on your ketogenic diet goals as well as keeping you in a positive mood while your body continues to burn fat (bringing you closer to your weight loss goals).

Caffeine helps to achieve weight loss goals by enhancing the breakdown of your body's fat, making it a great weight loss supplement to utilize while on the ketogenic diet.

Fiber: Most of the fiber that you will naturally consume while on the ketogenic diet is going to come from your vegetables, primarily from leafy green vegetables and broccoli (low carbohydrate vegetables that are also high in fiber, PERFECT for the ketogenic diet). By taking on a diet that strives to eliminate sources of carbohydrates such as grains, rice, pasta, and bread; you may be inadvertently eliminating the majority of your fiber intake as well (which is why it is essential to increase your consumption of broccoli and leafy green vegetables). Don't like leafy greens or broccoli? No problem, you can use a fiber supplement to make sure that you are still obtaining adequate amounts of fiber while on the ketogenic diet. The benefits of fiber are many and include the promotion of a healthy gut, keeping you feeling full for an extended period of time between meals, and keeping you regular. When it comes to adding a fiber supplement to your ketogenic diet plans, be sure to check out the nutrition labels because some fiber supplements can also be pretty high in carbohydrates (try to find a fiber supplement with a lower carb count). A great fiber supplement to pair with your ketogenic diet plans is Fiber 3 (produced by Now Nutrition) because it has a low carbohydrate content and relatively high-fat content. If you are not consuming enough fiber in your diet (either by regular food consumption or due to the lack of a fiber supplement), you make experience problems in the bathroom that can range from going too often or not being able to go at all. To avoid these unpleasant habits, be sure to find a good fiber supplement to add to your ketogenic diet plans.

Chapter 5:

Ketogenic Diet Recipes for Beginners

Smoothie Recipes

Chocolate Coconut Smoothie

Coconut Milk (1 Can Full Fat, Not Reduced)

Frozen Cherries (1 Cup)

.50 Ripe Avocado

Cacao Powder (.25 Cup)

Turmeric (.25 Tsp.)

*Filtered Water and Ice Cubes as needed

1. In a blender combine the following ingredients: coconut milk, frozen cherries, avocado, cacao powder, and turmeric. Blend together well, then add filtered water and ice cubes as needed to bring smoothie to the desired consistency.

2. To increase the thickness of the smoothie, you can add the unused half of the avocado. Leftover smoothies can be safely stored in the refrigerator for up to 24 hours.

Ketogenic Red Smoothie

5 Strawberries (Rinsed, Tops Removed, Chopped)

3 Ice Cubes

Fresh Raspberries (.50 Cup)

Red Cabbage (1 Cup: Chopped)

.50 Red Bell Pepper (Rinsed, Top Removed, Seeds Removed, Chopped)

1 Roma Tomato (Rinsed and Chopped)

Cold Water (8 oz.)

1. Prep all of the ingredients listed above and then move them to a blender. Pulse ingredients together until the smoothie achieves your desired consistency.

2. Serve in a separate glass while still cold and enjoy! Leftover smoothies can be safely stored in the refrigerator for up to 24 hours.

Almond Kale Smoothie

Kale (2 Cups)

2 Brazil Nuts

10 Almonds

Unsweetened Coconut Milk (1 Cup)

Vanilla Whey Protein (2 Scoops)

Psyllium Seeds (1 Tbsp. Can Substitute Chia Seeds)

Potato Starch (1 Tablespoon)

1. Using a blender, combine the following ingredients: coconut milk, brazil nuts, almonds, and kale. Blend together thoroughly until completely smooth.

2. Next, combine the rest of the ingredients: vanilla whey protein, psyllium seeds or chia seeds, and potato starch. Blend until smoothie reaches desired consistency, moved the desired amount to separate glass and enjoy. Leftover smoothies can be safely stored in the refrigerator for up to 24 hours.

Breakfast Recipes

Ketogenic Breakfast Sausage

Ground Pork (1 lb.)

Cold Water (3 Tbsp.)

Coconut Oil (1 Tbsp.)

Sea Salt (1 Tsp.)

Black Pepper

(.50 Tsp.)

Dried Sage (.50 Tsp.)

Dried Thyme

(.25 Tsp.)

Dried Ginger (.25 Tsp.)

1. Place the ground pork in a bowl and set aside. In a different bowl mix together the following ingredients: water, sea salt, black pepper, sage, thyme, and ginger. Mix together well then pour mixture over the ground pork. Blend these ingredients together thoroughly.

2. Shape the mixture into 8 small sausage patties, then fry sausage patties in coconut oil using a nonstick skillet. Fry for 5 minutes on the first side, then flip and fry for an additional 3 minutes. Serve warm and enjoy!

Spinach & Feta Frittata

12 Eggs

Raw Breakfast Sausage (12 oz. Pork or Beef)

Frozen/Chopped Spinach (10 oz.; Thaw and Drain)

Crumbled Feta Cheese (.50 Cup Crumbled)

Heavy Cream (.50 Cup)

Unsweetened Almond Milk (.25 Cup)

Sea Salt (.50 Tsp.)

Ground Nutmeg (.25 Tsp.)

Black Pepper (.25 Tsp.)

1. Preheat your home's oven (375 degrees Fahrenheit). Break the raw sausage up into significantly smaller pieces and leave in a clean bowl. Break up the spinach (thawed and drained) into the same bowl as the breakfast sausage pieces. Sprinkle crumbled feta cheese over the sausage and spinach mixture, toss until well combined.

2. Lightly grease a 13x9 baking dish with coconut oil or nonstick spray. Then spread previously made the mixture in the casserole dish, try to make sure it is evenly spread.

3. Using a different (preferably large) bowl, thoroughly combine the following ingredients: 12 eggs, black pepper, heavy cream, sea salt, almond milk, and nutmeg. Gently pour these mixed ingredients over the sausage mixture into the glass dish.

4. Bake in the prepared oven for 50 minutes or until it has fully set. Serve warm and enjoy!

Ketogenic Cream Cheese Pancakes

2 Eggs

Organic Cream Cheese (2 oz.; Non-Organic is OK also)

Coconut Flour (1 Tbsp.)

1 Packet of Stevia (Recommended: Stevia In The Raw)

Cinnamon (.50 Tsp.)

1. Combine all of the above-listed ingredients in a medium mixing bowl. Then, lightly grease a skillet with coconut oil or butter and allow the pan to heat up on medium heat.

2. Pour and cook the batter as you would with "normal" pancakes, allowing them to cook almost the whole way on one side before flipping. You can dress these in butter or sugar-free maple syrup, enjoy!

Spaghetti Squash Breakfast Casserole

1 Large Spaghetti Squash (Cut in half lengthwise, remove seeds)

2 Garlic Cloves (Minced)

4 Eggs

Onion (1 Cup Diced)

Diced Tomatoes (.50 Cup)

Italian Salami (3 oz. Sliced Thin)

Kalamata Olives (.50 Cup Halved)

Butter (4 Tbsp.)

Sea Salt

Black Pepper

Italian Seasoning (.50 Tsp.)

1. Preheat your home's oven (400 degrees Fahrenheit). Put both halves of the spaghetti squash with the cut side up on a baking tray. Spread 1 tablespoon of butter over each half, then sprinkle each with black pepper and sea salt. Bake these for 50 minutes in the oven.

2. In a nonstick pan or skillet, melt the remaining butter. After the butter has melted add in pepper, sea salt, onions, and garlic. Allow the onions to begin caramelization (they should take on an opaque appearance and change texture) and then add in the thin sliced salami and tomatoes. Sautee these ingredients for 10 minutes before adding in the Kalamata olives.

3. After the spaghetti squash has had a chance to finish roasting, remove the meat from each half using a fork, discard the skin and mix the flesh with the previously prepared onion mixture.

4. Use a tablespoon to create four wells or pockets in the skillet's mixture, then crack a single egg into each well. Relocate skillet to prepared oven and bake until the egg whites are completely cooked (cooking time will vary between 4-7 minutes).

5. Sprinkle with fresh parsley as a garnish, serve warm, and enjoy!

Dinner Recipes

Chicken Zucchini Pasta

Zucchini (2 Pounds)

Scallions (2)

Garlic (2 Cloves)

Mint Leaves (8; Fresh)

Pistachios (.25 Cup)

Lemon Juice (1 Tbsp.)

Boneless/Skinless Chicken Breast (4)

Sea Salt (1.5 Tbsp.)

Extra-Virgin Olive Oil (2 Tbsp.)

Ground Cumin (.25 Tsp.)

Black Pepper (.75 Tsp.)

1. Begin cooking this recipe by prepping the zucchini noodles (slice thin or spiralize if possible). After the zucchini has been transformed into noodles, toss them in a colander with the sea salt to lightly coat the strands. Leave the colander in your empty sink to drain while continuing with the rest of the recipe.

2. Slice the boneless/skinless chicken breasts into evenly sized strips. Place 1 Tbsp. of the olive oil in a pan to heat over medium/high heat on the stovetop. Gently transfer the chicken breast strips into the hot oil, seasoning lightly with black pepper and sea salt as they cook. Cook the chicken breast

strips (lightly coated in the olive oil) for three minutes on each side. Allow the chicken breast strips to cook for two minutes more until they are sizzling and browned on each side. Once finished, move breast strips to a plate and cover (loosely) with a single sheet of aluminum foil.

3. Use a small bowl to collect minced (preferably fresh) mint leaves, chopped pistachios, and scallions (thinly sliced). Pour the lemon juice over these three ingredients and stir together using a dinner fork.

4. Utilize a different bowl to combine together olive oil, ground cumin, crushed (and peeled) garlic, and black pepper. Mix together.

5. Use a medium-sized skillet set over medium/high heat on your home's stovetop to sauté the zucchini noodles for 2-3 minutes (until you gain a tender consistency). Pour the garlic seasoning mixture into the pan and stir to coat the noodles, cooking for about 20 seconds more. Remove from heat and top the zucchini noodles with chicken as well as a pistachio-mint combination. Toss to thoroughly combine if desired. Serve while all ingredients are still warm and enjoy!

Keto Taco Cups

Colby Jack Cheese (6 Slices)

Jalapeno (.50, Finely Diced)

Roma Tomatoes (2)

Lime Juice (From 1 Lime)

Red Onion (3 Tbsp./ Diced)

Cilantro (3 Tbsp.)

Ground Beef (.50 lb.)

1. Begin by preheating your home's oven to 375 degrees Fahrenheit. Use parchment to line a standard baking sheet, and then place each of the individual cheese slices to the sheet (leaving a few inches between each).

2. Using the previously heated oven, bake the cheese slices for an estimated five minutes (they should appear slightly browned at the edges and "bubbly"). After removing from the hot oven, allow the cheese slices to cool for a few minutes before carefully placing one in each muffin tin to form a cup-like shape (then allow to finish cooling while in the muffin tins).

3. Using a clean (medium/large) bowl to combine each of the following ingredients: cilantro, lime juice, roma tomatoes, jalapeno, and onions. Cover using cling-wrap (or aluminum foil) and transfer the bowl containing combined ingredients to the fridge to chill for an estimated thirty minutes.

4. Brown the ground beef in a clean skillet set on a stovetop over medium/high heat. Once the ground beef has been thoroughly browned, but not overcooked, remove the skillet from the stovetop's heat and drain the meat. Leave to cool slightly in the skillet while waiting for the salsa to finish cooling.

5. Assemble each of the taco cups using the previously made cheese cups, ground beef, and chilled salsa. You may top the keto taco cups with sour cream if desired, enjoy!

Garlic Butter Steak Strips

Garlic (6 Cloves)

Skirt Steak (1.5 lbs./ Trimmed/ Quartered)

Unsalted Butter (4 Tbsp.)

Canola Oil (2 Tbsp.)

Fresh Parsley (1 Tbsp./ Chopped)

Sea Salt

Ground (Black) Pepper

1. Begin by seasoning the four trips of steak (generously) using ground black pepper and sea salt. Heat up the canola oil using a medium/large skillet placed over high heat on your kitchen's stovetop. After the canola oil has had time to become hot, transfer the steak to the skillet to brown both sides well using the heated oil (3 minutes for each side if medium rare is desired). Allow the browned steak strips to rest on a clean plate while preparing the garlic butter sauce.

2. Use a new small/medium skillet to prepare the garlic butter sauce. Move this skillet over low heat on the stovetop and use this to melt down the butter to a consistent liquid. Once you have completely melted the butter, add the minced garlic and swirl while cooking for an estimated four minutes. Use sea salt to season the garlic butter sauce lightly.

3. Place the steak strips on individual plates to serve (or serve over zucchini pasta if desired), and gently spoon the previously made garlic butter sauce over the steak strips. Serve while warm, sprinkle with fresh parsley and enjoy!

Shrimp & Zucchini Pasta

Zucchini (2)

Lemon (1; Zest and Juice Only)

Shrimp (.75 lbs. / Peeled + Deveined)

Olive Oil (1 Tbsp.)

Garlic (4 Cloves, Minced)

Red Pepper Flakes

Ground Black Pepper

Sea Salt

Parsley (Fresh, Chopped)

1. Use a moderate setting to spiralize both zucchini to produce zucchini noodles. Move the prepared zucchini noodles aside to utilize later on in the recipe.

2. Use a clean skillet set over medium/high heat to heat the olive oil, lemon zest, and lemon juice together. Once these ingredients and the skillet are hot, add the prepared shrimp to the pan. Allow the shrimp to cook for roughly one minute on each side. Once the shrimp has cooked on each side, gently mix in the minced garlic as well as the red pepper flakes. Allow all ingredients to cook together for one more minute.

3. Be sure that you have allowed the shrimp, pepper flakes, and garlic to cook together for at least one minute, then transfer the previously made zucchini noodles into the pan with these ingredients. Use a clean pair of tongs to toss all

ingredients together well for three minutes so that the ingredients cook together as they are mixed.

4. Use ground black pepper and sea salt to season the entire dish to taste. Garnish by gently sprinkling freshly chopped parsley over the dish, serve while warm and enjoy!

Snack Recipes

Ketogenic Cookie Snack Bars

Coconut Butter (.75 Cup)

Apple Sauce (.24 Cup)

Sea Salt (.25 Tsp.)

Sesame Seeds (1.25 Cups)

Cinnamon (.50 Tsp.)

Vanilla Extract (.50 Tsp.)

1. Begin by preheating your home's oven to 350 degrees Fahrenheit. Use a medium/large-sized bowl to combine each of the following ingredients: sea salt, coconut butter, vanilla extract, cinnamon, and applesauce. Use a tablespoon to mix these ingredients together to combine them together well.

2. Divide the mixture evenly between 16 silicone muffin molds and press them flat. Then transfer the silicone molds to the previously warmed oven on a clean baking sheet, bake for twelve minutes. Once baked, remove the tray from the oven's heat and leave the silicone molds to cool for twenty minutes before attempting to remove the snack bars from molds.

3. Once cooled, move the snack bars to the freezer for twenty minutes: this will help them to chill quickly and become firm. Remove from freezer and serve at warm temp.

Sugar-Free Keto Bars

Mixed Nuts & Seeds (1.5 Cups)

Shredded Coconut (.25 Cup)

Cocoa Nibs (2 Tbsp.)

Coconut Oil (.25 Cup)

Almond Butter (4 Tbsp.)

Vanilla (1 Tsp.)

Cinnamon (2 Tsp.)

Sea Salt (.25 Tsp.)

Eggs (2)

1. After measuring and preparing all of the above ingredients, transfer all ingredients to an empty and clean blender. Pulse the blender four or five times so that all ingredients have been combined but so that the nuts and seeds are not ground finely (coarsely chopped).

2. Pour the ingredient mixture into a (previously greased) baking dish. Bake the ingredients in the dish together at 350 degrees Fahrenheit for an estimated twenty minutes. Serve warm or at room temperature and enjoy!

Maple Pecan Breakfast Bars

Pecans (2 Cups Halved)

Almond Flour (1 Cup)

Coconut Oil

(.50 Cup)

Shredded Coconut (.50 Cup) (Unsweetened)

Golden Flaxseed Meal (.50 Cup)

Sugar-Free Maple Syrup (.25 Cup)

Liquid Sweetener (.25 Tsp.)

1. Preheat you household oven (350 degrees Fahrenheit), and bake the two cups of pecan halves for 8 minutes. Remove from oven and transfer the baked pecan halves to a Ziploc bag. Crush them into chunks or pecan pieces.

2. Use a large or medium-sized mixing bowl, combine the following ingredients: unsweetened shredded coconut, golden flaxseed meal, and almond flour. After these three ingredients have been thoroughly combined, mix in the crushed pecans.

3. Lastly, add the following ingredients to the mixture: liquid sweetener, sugar-free maple syrup, and coconut oil. Mix these ingredients together well to form a dough. Transfer the dough to a 11x7 baking dish and press the dough so that it evenly covers the bottom of the dish.

4. Relocate the casserole dish to oven to bake for 25 minutes (until the edges have browned lightly). Remove the dish from

the oven and cool for 15 minutes. Then refrigerate for one hour to ensure easy, clean cuts.

5. After one hour in the refrigerator, cut into 12 bars and place in an airtight container. Enjoy!

Ketogenic Lemon Pudding

4 Eggs (Separated)

Mascarpone Cheese (1 oz.)

Unsalted Butter (.25 Cup)

Cream of Tartar (.25 Tsp.)

Monk Fruit Extract (.25 Tsp.)

Lemon Extract (.50 Tsp.)

Lemon Flavored Stevia Drops (.50 Tsp.)

1. Use a medium saucepan to melt and combine the butter and mascarpone cheese. After these ingredients have melted together, whisk in the egg yolks. Continue cooking these ingredients on low heat and stir occasionally until it begins to form a custard consistency. Take away from heat, proceed by stirring in the remaining ingredients (lemon flavoring and sweeteners).

2. Use a separate bowl to beat together the cream of tartar and separated egg whites, then combine the two mixtures and continue beating for an additional two minutes. Chill before serving. Enjoy!

Cinnamon Orange Scones

2 Eggs

Coconut Flour (.50 Cup)

Heavy Whipping Cream (.33 Cup Cooled)

Butter (.25 Cup Unsalted, Chilled, Cubed)

Erythritol (.25 Cup)

Sugar-Free Maple Syrup (2 Tbsp.)

 Coconut Oil (2 Tbsp.)

Golden Flaxseed (1 Tbsp.)

Orange Zest (1 Tbsp.)

Ground Cinnamon (2 Tsp.)

Baking Powder (1.5 Tsp.)

Vanilla Extract (1 Tsp.)

Sweetener (.25 Tsp.; Stevia, Equal, Splenda)

Xanthan Gum (.25 Tsp.)

Sea Salt (.25 Tsp.)

1. Preheat your home's oven (400 degrees Fahrenheit). Use a clean bowl to combine the following ingredients: orange zest, coconut oil, golden flaxseed, sea salt, baking powder, and 7 tablespoons of coconut flour.

2. Mix the ingredients previously listed together thoroughly before combining the cubes of chilled butter. Use a fork to be sure the butter is well incorporated into the mixture.

3. In a different bowl than previously used, combine the following ingredients: eggs, erythritol, and liquid sweetener. Once these ingredients are combined, and the eggs are light in color, add the following ingredients: sugar-free maple syrup, heavy whipping cream, and vanilla extract. Continue mixing these ingredients until the cream thickens.

4. Combine the two mixtures in a bowl (save 2 tablespoons of cream mixture for later) and add the xanthan gum and coconut flour, and knead the mixture to form a dough. Add the ground cinnamon and continue kneading until the cinnamon is well mixed into the ball of dough. Mold this dough to form a flat circle that is about an inch thick.

5. Cut the circle of dough into 8 triangular slices, like you would cut a pizza into 8 slices. Place the dough slices onto a cookie sheet (line sheet with wax paper or parchment). Use a brush to coat the slices with the leftover cream mixture and sprinkle the tops with cinnamon.

6. Bake the scones for 15-18 minutes, then allow them to cool for 20-25 minutes once removed from the oven. Serve warm and enjoy!

Ketogenic Cloud Bread

4 Eggs

Light Cream Cheese (4 Tbsp. Softened)

1 Packet Granular Sweetener

Cream of Tartar (.50 Tsp.)

Sea Salt

1. Preheat your home's oven (350 degrees Fahrenheit) and prepare two baking trays with parchment paper or wax paper.

2. Use two separate mixing bowls to separate egg yolks and egg whites, then add the cream of tartar to the mixing bowl containing the egg whites. Use an electric mixer to beat for 3-5 minutes until the egg whites stiffen.

3. Add the following ingredients to the mixing bowl containing the egg yolks: granular sweetener, sea salt, and cream cheese. Whisk the egg yolk mixture together thoroughly, then gently fold this mixture in with the egg whites mixture. Your prepared batter should appear fluffy.

4. Scoop the batter onto the baking sheets, placing about 6 scoops of batter evenly spread on each (they will spread as they bake). Bake the baking sheets for 20-21 minutes, switch the position of the trays halfway through. Once done, allow the bread to cool completely before removing from the baking trays and serving. Enjoy!

Conclusion

Thank you again for downloading this book!

I hope this book was able to help you to gain a better understanding of what the ketogenic diet is, how it works, and the various health benefits that it can offer to you.

The next step is to use the information provided to begin your own ketogenic diet experience so that you may experience better health and wellness. Whether your goals are to maintain healthy cholesterol levels, lower your blood pressure, or to lose weight; the ketogenic diet can help you to achieve those goals! By downloading and reading this eBook, we hope you are one step closer to achieving those goals and having a positive experience with the ketogenic diet. Remember that no matter the issue with the ketogenic diet, there is almost always a solution that can be offered by simply tweaking your daily dietary habits.

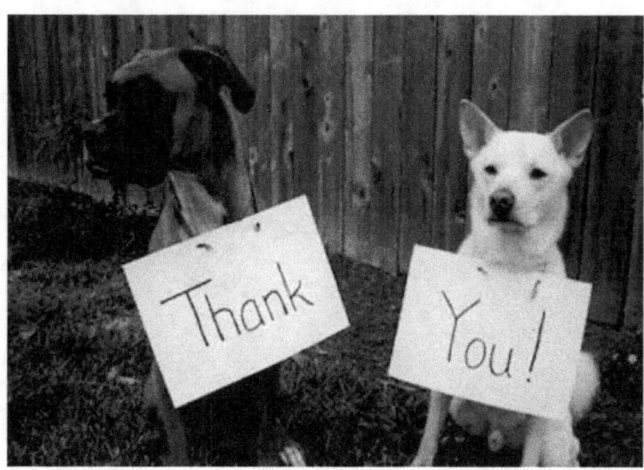

Finally, if you enjoyed this book, then I'd like to ask you for a favor, would you be kind enough to leave a review for this book on Amazon? It'd be greatly appreciated!

Thank you and good luck!